Table of Contents

Introduction 5
   Importance of Good Sleep 5
   Purpose of the Book 7
   Overview of Comparison Methods 9

Chapter 1: Sleep Trackers 11
   How They Work and What They Track 11
   Pros and Cons 13
   Popular Brands 16

Chapter 2: Smart Mattresses 19
   How They Work and What They Offer 19
   Pros and Cons 22
   Popular Mattresses 25

Chapter 3: Sleep Apps 27
   How They Work and What They Offer 27
   Pros and Cons 29
   Popular Apps 32

Chapter 4: White Noise Machines 34
   How They Work and What They Offer 34
   Pros and Cons 36
   Popular Machines 38

Chapter 5: Light Therapy Devices 40
   How They Work and What They Offer 40
   Pros and Cons 42

Popular Devices *44*

Chapter 6: Smart Pillows 47
How They Work and What They Offer *47*

Pros and Cons *49*

Popular Pillows.. *51*

Chapter 7: Sleep Sound Machines 54
How They Work and What They Offer *54*

Pros and Cons *58*

Popular Machines... *61*

Chapter 8: Comparing and Contrasting Methods .. 66
Summary of Pros and Cons....................................*66*

Criteria for Comparison...................................... *72*

Recommendations for Different Needs.....................*75*

Conclusion 78
Recap of Importance of Good Sleep *78*

Final Thoughts and Recommendations *80*

Potential References.. 83

Copyright © 2023 by Herman Strange (Author)

All rights reserved. This book or any portion thereof may not be reproduced or used in any manner whatsoever without the express written permission of the publisher except for the use of brief quotations in a book review.

This book is copyright protected. This is only for personal use. You cannot amend, distributor, sell, use, quote or paraphrase any part or the content within this book without the consent of the author. Please note the information contained within this document is for educational and entertainment purposes only. Every attempt has been made to provide accurate, up to date and reliable complete information. No warranties of any kind are expressed or implied.

Readers acknowledge that the author is not engaging in the rendering of legal, financial, medical or professional advice. The content of this book has been derived from various sources. Please consult a licensed professional before attempting any techniques outlined in this book.

By reading this document, the readers agree that under no circumstances are the author responsible for any losses, direct or indirect, which are incurred as a result of the use of information contained within this document, including but not limited to errors, omissions or inaccuracies.

Thank you very much for reading this book.

Title: Sleeping for Health-How to Optimize Your Sleep for Physical and Mental Well-being
Subtitle: Tips and Tricks for Achieving Better Sleep

Series: Healthy Habits for Life: Building Sustainable Habits for Optimal Health and Wellness
Author: Serenity Tanner

Introduction
Importance of Good Sleep

Sleep is an essential part of our lives and a crucial aspect of our overall health and wellbeing. We spend roughly one-third of our lives sleeping, and the quality of our sleep can significantly impact our physical and mental health. Good quality sleep is crucial to help our body and mind rest, recover, and rejuvenate.

Poor sleep quality has been linked to a variety of health problems, such as obesity, diabetes, heart disease, high blood pressure, and even depression and anxiety. Additionally, lack of sleep can impact our productivity, cognitive function, and overall mood.

While we all know that sleep is important, many of us often underestimate its significance, and our busy lives can sometimes make it challenging to get the recommended amount of sleep each night. It's essential to prioritize sleep and create a healthy sleep routine to ensure we get the most out of our sleep.

In this book, we will discuss various methods and devices that can help you track and improve your sleep quality. With these tools, you can gain insight into your sleep patterns, identify potential issues, and make necessary changes to improve the quality of your sleep. By making sleep a priority and taking steps to improve your sleep quality, you can improve your overall health and wellbeing and get the most out of your waking hours.

Purpose of the Book

The primary purpose of this book is to provide readers with a comprehensive guide to sleep tracking methods and devices, which can help them improve the quality of their sleep. In today's fast-paced world, where many people struggle with stress, anxiety, and sleep disorders, it's essential to prioritize good quality sleep to maintain good health and wellbeing.

In this book, we will discuss various sleep tracking methods and devices, such as sleep trackers, smart mattresses, sleep apps, white noise machines, light therapy devices, smart pillows, and sleep sound machines. By exploring each of these methods in-depth, we aim to provide readers with the knowledge they need to choose the best method or combination of methods to suit their unique sleep needs.

The book will include information on how each method works, what it tracks or offers, and its pros and cons. Additionally, we will highlight popular brands and products in each category, as well as provide a summary of the criteria for comparison.

Our ultimate goal is to empower readers to take control of their sleep health by providing them with the tools they need to track, analyze and improve their sleep quality.

We believe that by understanding the importance of good sleep and taking steps to improve it, readers can improve their overall health and wellbeing, reduce stress and anxiety, and live a more productive, fulfilling life.

Whether you're struggling with sleep problems, looking to optimize your sleep routine, or just interested in learning more about the latest sleep tracking methods and devices, this book is designed to provide you with the knowledge and tools you need to achieve your sleep goals.

Overview of Comparison Methods

With so many sleep tracking methods and devices available on the market, it can be challenging to determine which ones will work best for your needs. In this book, we aim to provide a comprehensive overview of the different sleep tracking methods and devices, highlighting their features, benefits, and potential drawbacks to help readers make an informed decision.

The comparison will be based on various criteria, including accuracy, ease of use, price, data tracking, and sleep analysis features. We will also consider the level of customization, durability, and compatibility with other devices.

To compare the different methods, we will analyze each one in-depth and provide a detailed overview of how it works and what it offers. For example, we will explore how sleep trackers work, the different types of sensors they use, and the data they track, including sleep duration, stages, and patterns.

We will also discuss the pros and cons of each method, such as the accuracy of sleep tracking, the level of comfort, the ease of use, the type of data provided, and the cost of the device.

By providing a detailed comparison of each method, we aim to help readers determine which method or combination of methods will be most effective for their sleep needs. Additionally, we will provide recommendations for different needs, such as the best methods for individuals with sleep disorders, for those who travel frequently, or for those who are looking for a budget-friendly option.

Ultimately, our goal is to provide readers with the information they need to make an informed decision about the best sleep tracking methods and devices to improve their sleep quality. By understanding the different options available, readers can choose the best method for their unique needs, and take control of their sleep health.

Chapter 1: Sleep Trackers
How They Work and What They Track

Sleep trackers are one of the most popular methods of sleep tracking, and they work by using sensors to track various sleep-related data. The sensors can be embedded in a device that is worn on the wrist or attached to clothing, or they can be part of a bed sensor that is placed under the mattress.

The sensors used in sleep trackers are typically accelerometers and/or gyroscopes, which track movements and vibrations during the night. By analyzing these movements and vibrations, the sleep tracker can determine when you are awake, in light sleep, in deep sleep, or in REM sleep.

In addition to tracking sleep stages, sleep trackers can also track other sleep-related data, such as the number of times you wake up during the night, the duration of sleep, the time it takes to fall asleep, and the overall sleep quality. Many sleep trackers also include features such as heart rate tracking and temperature monitoring, which can provide additional insight into your sleep patterns.

Some sleep trackers can also be synced with a smartphone app or other devices to provide a more comprehensive overview of your sleep data. This can include visualizations of your sleep patterns, sleep quality scores, and personalized insights based on your sleep data.

However, it's important to note that not all sleep trackers are equally accurate. Some studies have found that certain sleep trackers can overestimate or underestimate sleep duration and sleep stages, which can impact the accuracy of the data. Additionally, the accuracy of sleep trackers can be affected by factors such as device placement, user movements during the night, and the type of sleep disorder being tracked.

In summary, sleep trackers work by using sensors to track sleep-related data, including sleep stages, sleep quality, and other metrics such as heart rate and temperature. The data can be visualized and analyzed to provide insights into your sleep patterns, and many sleep trackers can be synced with other devices to provide a more comprehensive overview of your sleep data. However, it's important to be aware of the potential limitations of sleep trackers, including their accuracy and the impact of external factors.

Pros and Cons

Sleep trackers can be a useful tool for people who are interested in improving their sleep quality. Here are some of the pros and cons of using a sleep tracker:

Pros:

1. Provides objective data: A sleep tracker can provide objective data about your sleep patterns, including sleep duration, sleep stages, and other sleep-related metrics. This can be especially useful for people who have trouble sleeping or who want to optimize their sleep quality.

2. Identifies sleep issues: By tracking sleep data over time, a sleep tracker can help you identify patterns and potential issues with your sleep. For example, if you consistently have trouble falling asleep, the data from your sleep tracker can help you identify potential reasons for this and make changes to your sleep routine to improve it.

3. Offers personalized insights: Some sleep trackers come with personalized insights and recommendations based on your sleep data. These can help you identify areas for improvement and make changes to your sleep routine to optimize your sleep quality.

4. Provides motivation: Seeing progress over time can be motivating, and some sleep trackers offer features such as badges or rewards for achieving sleep-related goals. This can

help people stay motivated to make changes and improve their sleep quality.

Cons:

1. Cost: Sleep trackers can be expensive, with some models costing several hundred dollars. This may not be a feasible option for everyone.

2. Accuracy: While sleep trackers can provide useful data, their accuracy can vary. Some sleep trackers may overestimate or underestimate sleep stages or sleep duration, which can impact the usefulness of the data.

3. User error: The accuracy of sleep trackers can be affected by user error, such as forgetting to wear the device or not placing it in the right location. This can impact the accuracy of the data and the usefulness of the sleep tracker.

4. Can be distracting: Some people may find that the act of tracking their sleep using a device can be distracting or even anxiety-provoking. This can make it harder to fall asleep and impact the overall sleep quality.

In summary, sleep trackers can be a useful tool for improving sleep quality, providing objective data, identifying sleep issues, offering personalized insights, and providing motivation. However, they can be expensive, their accuracy can vary, they can be affected by user error, and they can be distracting or anxiety-provoking for some people. It's important to carefully consider the pros and cons of using a sleep tracker before investing in one.

Popular Brands

When it comes to sleep trackers, there are many brands and models to choose from. Here are some of the most popular brands of sleep trackers and their features:

1. Fitbit: Fitbit is a popular brand of sleep tracker that offers a range of models at different price points. Some of their sleep tracking features include tracking sleep stages, sleep duration, and sleep quality. They also offer personalized insights and recommendations based on sleep data.

2. Garmin: Garmin is another popular brand of sleep tracker that offers a range of models at different price points. Some of their sleep tracking features include tracking sleep stages, sleep duration, and sleep quality. They also offer personalized insights and recommendations based on sleep data.

3. Withings: Withings is a brand of sleep tracker that offers a variety of models, including a smartwatch that can track sleep. Some of their sleep tracking features include tracking sleep stages, sleep duration, and sleep quality. They also offer personalized insights and recommendations based on sleep data.

4. Oura: Oura is a sleep tracker that comes in the form of a ring. Some of its sleep tracking features include tracking

sleep stages, sleep duration, and sleep quality. It also offers personalized insights and recommendations based on sleep data.

5. SleepScore Labs: SleepScore Labs offers a sleep tracker that works by placing a small device under your mattress. It tracks sleep stages, sleep duration, and sleep quality, and provides personalized insights and recommendations based on sleep data.

6. Apple Watch: While not specifically marketed as a sleep tracker, the Apple Watch can track sleep stages, sleep duration, and sleep quality using third-party apps. It also offers personalized insights and recommendations based on sleep data.

7. Polar: Polar is a brand of sleep tracker that offers a range of models at different price points. Some of their sleep tracking features include tracking sleep stages, sleep duration, and sleep quality. They also offer personalized insights and recommendations based on sleep data.

It's important to note that these are just a few of the many sleep tracker brands and models available on the market. When choosing a sleep tracker, it's important to consider your budget, the features that are most important to you, and the level of accuracy and reliability you need.

Overall, sleep trackers can be a useful tool for improving sleep quality, but it's important to carefully consider the features and capabilities of different models before making a purchase. By doing so, you can choose a sleep tracker that is best suited to your individual needs and preferences.

Chapter 2: Smart Mattresses
How They Work and What They Offer

How They Work

Smart mattresses are designed to use technology to help people achieve better sleep. They typically include a variety of sensors and other features that can track your sleep, adjust the mattress to your preferred level of firmness, and even wake you up at the best possible time based on your sleep cycle. Here are some of the key components and features of smart mattresses:

1. Sensors: Smart mattresses typically use a variety of sensors to track your sleep, including accelerometers, pressure sensors, and temperature sensors. These sensors can track your movements, heart rate, and other vital signs to provide a comprehensive picture of your sleep quality.

2. Smart controls: Many smart mattresses come with a control panel or smartphone app that allows you to adjust the firmness and other settings of the mattress. This can be particularly helpful for couples who have different preferences for firmness.

3. Heating and cooling: Some smart mattresses come with heating and cooling features that can adjust the temperature of the bed based on your preferences. This can

be particularly helpful for people who struggle with night sweats or other temperature-related sleep issues.

4. Sleep tracking: Smart mattresses can track your sleep patterns and provide detailed reports on your sleep quality. This can help you identify any issues that may be affecting your sleep, such as snoring or sleep apnea.

What They Offer

Smart mattresses offer a variety of benefits that can help people achieve better sleep. Here are some of the main benefits of smart mattresses:

1. Personalized support: Smart mattresses can be customized to your preferred level of firmness, providing personalized support that can help relieve pressure points and reduce pain.

2. Temperature control: Smart mattresses with heating and cooling features can help regulate your body temperature for optimal sleep.

3. Sleep tracking: Smart mattresses can provide detailed information on your sleep patterns, which can help you identify any issues that may be affecting your sleep.

4. Smart alarms: Some smart mattresses can be programmed to wake you up at the best possible time based on your sleep cycle. This can help you wake up feeling more refreshed and alert.

5. Smart home integration: Some smart mattresses can be integrated with other smart home devices, such as lights and thermostats, to create a more personalized sleep environment.

Overall, smart mattresses can offer a range of benefits for people looking to improve their sleep quality. By using advanced technology to track your sleep and adjust the mattress to your preferred level of firmness, these mattresses can help you achieve a more restful and rejuvenating night's sleep.

Pros and Cons

Smart mattresses are a relatively new type of sleep technology that can offer a range of benefits for improving sleep. However, like any other sleep-tracking device, there are also some potential drawbacks to consider. In this section, we'll explore the pros and cons of using a smart mattress for sleep tracking and improvement.

Pros:

1. Comprehensive Sleep Tracking: Smart mattresses use a range of sensors to track a wide variety of sleep-related data, including body movements, heart rate, breathing, and more. This level of detail can provide users with a comprehensive understanding of their sleep patterns, which can be useful for identifying areas that need improvement.

2. Customized Sleep Recommendations: Based on the data collected, some smart mattresses are equipped with machine learning algorithms that can provide customized recommendations for improving sleep quality. For example, the mattress might suggest adjusting the room temperature or changing the user's sleep position.

3. Adjustable Firmness: Many smart mattresses come with adjustable firmness settings that can be customized to the user's preferences. This feature can be particularly

helpful for people with back or joint pain who need a specific level of support to feel comfortable.

4. Connected Home Integration: Smart mattresses can integrate with other smart home devices to create a more streamlined sleep experience. For example, the mattress might automatically adjust the temperature or turn off the lights when the user goes to bed.

Cons:

1. High Cost: Smart mattresses are often more expensive than traditional mattresses, and they can come with additional fees for sleep tracking software or maintenance. This cost might be prohibitive for some users.

2. Limited Compatibility: Smart mattresses may not be compatible with all bed frames or sleep positions, which could limit their usefulness for some users.

3. Learning Curve: Some users may find that the process of setting up and using a smart mattress is more complicated than traditional sleep-tracking methods. Additionally, because the mattress collects data automatically, users may need to take steps to ensure that their data is secure and protected.

4. Potential for Malfunctions: Like any technology, smart mattresses can malfunction or break down, which could require expensive repairs or replacements.

Overall, smart mattresses can offer a range of benefits for improving sleep quality, but they may not be the best fit for everyone. It's important to weigh the pros and cons carefully before making a decision.

Popular Mattresses

In recent years, smart mattresses have gained popularity among people looking to improve their sleep. These mattresses use advanced technology to track your sleep and offer features to improve it. Here are some popular smart mattresses on the market:

1. Eight Sleep Pod: The Eight Sleep Pod is a high-tech mattress that uses a variety of sensors to track your sleep. It offers personalized temperature control, can wake you up with a gentle vibration, and can integrate with other smart home devices.

2. Sleep Number 360: The Sleep Number 360 uses sensors to adjust the firmness of the mattress based on your sleeping position. It also has a variety of other features, including a foot warmer and adjustable headrest.

3. The Pod by Eight Sleep: The Pod is another offering from Eight Sleep that uses advanced temperature control to help you sleep better. It can also track your sleep and offer insights into how to improve it.

4. Nectar: The Nectar mattress has a sleep tracking feature that can integrate with a smartphone app. It also offers a 365-night trial and lifetime warranty.

5. Tempur-Pedic: Tempur-Pedic mattresses have long been popular for their comfortable memory foam technology.

They also offer a range of smart features, including a sleep tracker, adjustable firmness, and cooling technology.

6. Beautyrest Sleeptracker: The Beautyrest Sleeptracker is a mattress topper that uses sensors to track your sleep. It can integrate with Amazon's Alexa to provide insights and advice on how to improve your sleep.

Each of these mattresses offers unique features and benefits, but they also come with some drawbacks. For example, some people may find the high-tech features overwhelming or difficult to use, while others may not see the value in spending extra money on a smart mattress. As with any sleep product, it's important to carefully consider your own needs and preferences before making a purchase.

Chapter 3: Sleep Apps
How They Work and What They Offer

Sleep apps are designed to help you track and monitor your sleep using your smartphone or other mobile device. They typically use the sensors built into your phone to track movement and sound during the night, providing data that can be used to analyze your sleep quality. Here is an overview of how sleep apps work and what they offer:

1. Sleep Tracking: The main feature of sleep apps is tracking your sleep patterns. Many apps use your phone's accelerometer to detect movement during the night, which can help determine how long you slept, how often you woke up, and how long it took you to fall asleep.

2. Sleep Stages: Some sleep apps can track the different stages of sleep, such as deep sleep, light sleep, and REM sleep. By tracking these stages, the app can provide more detailed insights into your sleep quality and help you identify areas for improvement.

3. Smart Alarms: Many sleep apps offer a smart alarm feature that uses your sleep data to wake you up at the optimal time, when you are in a light sleep stage. This can help you feel more refreshed and energized in the morning.

4. Sleep Environment: Some sleep apps can also track environmental factors that may impact your sleep, such as

noise levels and room temperature. This information can help you make adjustments to your sleeping environment to create a more comfortable and restful space.

5. Sleep Tips and Education: Some sleep apps also offer tips and educational resources to help you improve your sleep habits. This may include information on healthy sleep habits, relaxation techniques, and advice on how to establish a regular sleep schedule.

Overall, sleep apps offer a convenient and accessible way to track your sleep and gain insights into your sleep quality. However, it's important to note that sleep apps can have limitations, such as the accuracy of the data collected, and may not be a substitute for a professional medical diagnosis. It's also important to choose a reputable sleep app from a trusted source and carefully consider the app's privacy policy to ensure that your personal information is protected.

Pros and Cons

Sleep apps are an increasingly popular way to track and improve sleep. However, like any other method of sleep tracking, sleep apps have their pros and cons. In this section, we will discuss the advantages and disadvantages of sleep apps.

Pros:

1. Convenient and easy to use: Sleep apps are very convenient and easy to use. They are available on smartphones and can be used anywhere and at any time. All you need to do is download the app, set it up, and place your phone on your nightstand.

2. Provides useful information: Sleep apps can provide useful information about your sleep patterns. They can track the duration and quality of your sleep, as well as provide information on factors that may be affecting your sleep.

3. Offers personalized insights: Sleep apps can offer personalized insights into your sleep patterns. They can provide you with recommendations based on your sleep data and help you identify patterns and trends that may be affecting your sleep.

4. Cost-effective: Sleep apps are generally cost-effective. Most sleep apps are free or available at a low cost,

making them an affordable way to track and improve your sleep.

5. A wide variety of apps to choose from: There is a wide variety of sleep apps available, each offering different features and functions. This means that you can choose the app that best suits your needs and preferences.

Cons:

1. Accuracy: Sleep apps may not be as accurate as other methods of sleep tracking, such as sleep trackers or smart mattresses. They rely on sensors within your smartphone to detect movement and sound, which may not be as reliable as other methods.

2. Phone dependency: Sleep apps require the use of your smartphone, which means that you must have your phone with you in bed. This can be a problem for some people who prefer to disconnect from their phone at night.

3. Potential for app-related stress: Sleep apps may cause stress or anxiety in some users. For example, if the app shows that you did not get enough sleep, this may cause you to worry and make it harder to fall asleep the next night.

4. Battery drain: Sleep apps can drain your phone's battery quickly, which can be a problem if you need your phone for other purposes.

5. Lack of regulation: Sleep apps are not regulated by any governing body, which means that there is no standard for accuracy or reliability. This means that the quality of sleep apps can vary widely.

Overall, sleep apps can be a useful tool for tracking and improving your sleep. However, they do have their limitations, and it is important to carefully consider the pros and cons before choosing a sleep app to use.

Popular Apps

When it comes to sleep apps, there are a multitude of options available, each with their own unique features and benefits. Here are a few of the most popular sleep apps on the market today:

1. Sleep Cycle Sleep Cycle is one of the most well-known sleep tracking apps, and for good reason. The app uses your phone's accelerometer to track your movements and determine which stage of sleep you're in. It then wakes you up during your lightest stage of sleep, which can help you feel more rested and refreshed. Sleep Cycle also offers in-app sleep notes, sleep statistics, and a variety of soothing wake-up sounds.

2. Calm Calm is a popular app for meditation and relaxation, but it also offers a range of features for sleep. The app includes sleep stories, guided meditations, and soothing sounds to help you relax and fall asleep. Calm also offers a feature called "Sleep Stories," which are narrated by well-known celebrities and designed to help you drift off to sleep.

3. Headspace Headspace is another popular meditation app that also offers features for sleep. The app offers guided meditations designed to help you relax and fall asleep, as well as breathing exercises and a variety of sleep sounds. One unique feature of Headspace is "Sleepcasts,"

which are audio experiences designed to transport you to a peaceful place and help you fall asleep.

4. Pillow Pillow is a comprehensive sleep tracking app that uses your phone's microphone to detect snoring, sleep talking, and other sounds during the night. The app also offers sleep stage analysis, sleep statistics, and a variety of wake-up sounds. One unique feature of Pillow is its "Smart Alarm," which wakes you up during your lightest stage of sleep, similar to Sleep Cycle.

5. White Noise White Noise is a popular app that offers a wide range of soothing sounds to help you relax and fall asleep. The app includes a variety of white noise sounds, as well as other ambient sounds like rain, waves, and wind. White Noise also offers a feature called "Mix Pad," which allows you to create custom soundscapes by combining different sounds.

These are just a few examples of the many sleep apps available today. Each app has its own unique features and benefits, so it's important to research and try out a few to find the one that works best for you.

Chapter 4: White Noise Machines
How They Work and What They Offer

White noise machines are designed to create a consistent background noise that helps to block out other distracting sounds and create a soothing environment conducive to sleep. They work by producing a sound that contains all frequencies at equal intensity, which can mask or drown out other sounds that might otherwise be disruptive to sleep.

White noise machines can produce a range of sounds, from pure white noise to different types of colored noise, such as pink noise, brown noise, and gray noise. Some machines also offer natural sounds like rainfall, ocean waves, or forest sounds. The user can choose the sound that is most relaxing or effective in blocking out unwanted noise.

One of the benefits of white noise machines is that they can help to create a consistent sleep environment, which is especially helpful for light sleepers or those who live in noisy areas. They can also be used to help babies or young children fall asleep and stay asleep, and can help shift workers sleep during the daytime.

However, there are some potential drawbacks to using white noise machines. Some people find the noise itself to be distracting or irritating, and may have difficulty falling asleep with it on. In addition, some machines can be quite loud, which may not be suitable for those who need a quiet environment to sleep.

Furthermore, prolonged exposure to loud noise, even white noise, can be harmful to hearing, so it is important to use white noise machines at a safe volume level. Additionally, some people may become reliant on white noise machines to sleep, which can make it difficult for them to fall asleep without the machine.

Overall, white noise machines can be an effective tool for promoting good sleep, but like any sleep aid, they have both advantages and disadvantages. It's important to weigh these factors carefully and consider whether a white noise machine is a good fit for your individual sleep needs.

Pros and Cons

White noise machines are commonly used to promote better sleep by providing a steady stream of white noise, which can help mask disruptive sounds and create a more peaceful sleeping environment. However, like any sleep aid, white noise machines have their pros and cons.

Pros:

1. Improved sleep quality: White noise machines can help improve sleep quality by masking disruptive sounds and creating a consistent background noise that can help lull the brain into a state of relaxation.

2. Reduced stress and anxiety: Many people find the consistent background noise created by a white noise machine to be soothing and calming, which can help reduce feelings of stress and anxiety.

3. Portable and easy to use: White noise machines are often small and portable, making them easy to take with you when traveling or moving from room to room.

4. Cost-effective: Many white noise machines are relatively inexpensive and can provide a cost-effective solution for people looking to improve their sleep.

Cons:

1. Can be distracting: While white noise can help mask disruptive sounds, it can also be distracting in and of itself, especially if it is too loud or too inconsistent.

2. May not work for everyone: While many people find white noise to be calming and helpful for sleep, it may not work for everyone. Some people may find it irritating or disruptive to their sleep.

3. May not address underlying sleep issues: While white noise machines can help create a more peaceful sleeping environment, they may not address underlying sleep issues such as sleep apnea or other sleep disorders.

4. Limited effectiveness: Some people may find that white noise machines are only effective for a limited period of time, and that they lose their effectiveness over time.

Despite these potential drawbacks, many people find that white noise machines can be an effective tool for improving their sleep quality. When used correctly and in conjunction with other healthy sleep habits, white noise machines can provide a cost-effective and easy-to-use solution for people looking to get a better night's sleep.

Popular Machines

Sure, here's some content for "Popular Machines" in Chapter 4 on White Noise Machines:

White noise machines have become a popular choice for those who have trouble sleeping. These devices emit a constant and soothing sound that can help drown out other noises and create a peaceful sleeping environment. Here are some of the popular white noise machines on the market:

1. Marpac Dohm Classic: The Marpac Dohm Classic is a mechanical white noise machine that produces a natural and consistent sound. It has two-speed options and is compact, making it easy to take on-the-go.

2. LectroFan: The LectroFan is an electronic white noise machine that offers a wide range of white noise and fan sounds. It has ten different fan sounds and ten different white noise sounds to choose from, making it highly customizable.

3. HoMedics SoundSpa: The HoMedics SoundSpa is a compact white noise machine that offers six different sound options. It includes white noise, rain, brook, ocean, thunder, and summer night sounds to choose from.

4. Adaptive Sound Technologies Sound+Sleep: The Adaptive Sound Technologies Sound+Sleep is an electronic white noise machine that has 10 different sound profiles to

choose from. These sound profiles are highly customizable and include natural sounds, such as ocean waves and rainfall, as well as abstract sounds, like "twinkle" and "swell."

5. Yogasleep Rohm: The Yogasleep Rohm is a compact and portable white noise machine that can be attached to a stroller or car seat. It offers three different sound options: bright white noise, deep white noise, and gentle surf.

All of these white noise machines have their own unique features, and the best one for you will depend on your personal preferences and needs. It's important to consider factors such as sound quality, portability, and ease of use when choosing a white noise machine.

Chapter 5: Light Therapy Devices
How They Work and What They Offer

Light therapy devices are designed to help regulate the body's natural sleep-wake cycle by mimicking the effects of natural sunlight. These devices emit bright light that is similar in color and intensity to natural sunlight, and they are often used to treat seasonal affective disorder (SAD) and other sleep-related conditions.

One of the primary mechanisms by which light therapy devices work is by stimulating the production of serotonin, a neurotransmitter that regulates mood and promotes wakefulness. Exposure to bright light in the morning can increase serotonin levels and help regulate the body's internal clock, which is responsible for setting the sleep-wake cycle.

Light therapy devices are available in a range of styles and designs, including light boxes, lamps, and wearable devices. Some devices are designed to be used in the morning, while others can be used throughout the day or even at night to help regulate the body's internal clock.

One of the main benefits of light therapy devices is their ability to regulate the body's internal clock, which can help improve sleep quality and promote wakefulness during the day. These devices can be particularly useful for individuals who work irregular schedules or who live in regions with limited sunlight, as they can help regulate the body's natural sleep-wake cycle.

However, there are also some potential drawbacks to using light therapy devices. One of the main concerns is the potential for overstimulation, which can lead to sleep disturbances and other negative side effects. Additionally, some individuals may experience headaches or other symptoms when exposed to bright light for extended periods of time.

Overall, the benefits of light therapy devices for sleep regulation appear to outweigh the potential risks, particularly for individuals who are struggling with sleep-related conditions such as SAD or insomnia. However, it is important to carefully follow the manufacturer's instructions and to speak with a healthcare provider before using these devices to ensure that they are safe and effective for your individual needs.

Some popular light therapy devices on the market include the Philips SmartSleep Light Therapy Lamp, the Verilux HappyLight Therapy Lamp, and the Circadian Optics Lumos 2.0 Light Therapy Lamp.

Pros and Cons

Light therapy devices are a relatively new entrant in the market of sleep aids, but they have gained popularity in recent years. Here are some of the pros and cons of using light therapy devices to improve your sleep:

Pros:

1. Regulating circadian rhythms: Light therapy devices can help regulate your circadian rhythms, which can lead to better sleep. They work by simulating natural light, which can help reset your body clock and improve sleep quality.

2. Natural and non-invasive: Light therapy devices are non-invasive and use natural light, making them a safe and drug-free option for those who want to improve their sleep.

3. Effective for sleep disorders: Light therapy has been found to be effective in treating sleep disorders such as insomnia, sleep apnea, and shift work disorder.

4. Convenient and easy to use: Light therapy devices are easy to use and can be integrated into your daily routine. They are also portable, which makes them convenient for people who travel frequently.

Cons:

1. Potential side effects: While light therapy is generally safe, some people may experience side effects such as headaches, eye strain, and nausea.

2. Requires consistency: To see the benefits of light therapy, you need to be consistent in using the device every day. This can be challenging for some people who have a busy schedule or who may forget to use the device regularly.

3. May not work for everyone: Light therapy may not be effective for everyone, especially those who have severe sleep disorders or who have other underlying health conditions.

4. Can be expensive: Light therapy devices can be expensive, especially those that offer more advanced features. This can make them less accessible for some people.

In summary, light therapy devices can be an effective and safe option for those who want to improve their sleep quality. However, they may not work for everyone, and consistency is important to see the benefits. It is essential to weigh the pros and cons before investing in a light therapy device.

Popular Devices

In recent years, light therapy has become a popular tool for addressing a variety of health issues, including sleep disorders. As a result, there are now a wide variety of light therapy devices on the market, each with their own unique features and benefits. In this section, we will discuss some of the most popular light therapy devices currently available.

1. Verilux HappyLight: The Verilux HappyLight is a popular light therapy device that is designed to simulate natural sunlight. It emits 10,000 lux of bright white light, which is intended to help regulate the body's circadian rhythm and improve mood. The HappyLight is also portable, making it easy to use at home or in the office.

2. Philips SmartSleep Wake-Up Light: The Philips SmartSleep Wake-Up Light is a unique light therapy device that is designed to help users wake up more naturally. It gradually increases the amount of light in the room over a period of 30 minutes, simulating a sunrise and helping the body adjust to a natural wake-up cycle. The Wake-Up Light also includes customizable alarm sounds and a snooze function.

3. Circadian Optics Lumine Light Therapy Lamp: The Circadian Optics Lumine Light Therapy Lamp is another popular light therapy device that is designed to mimic

natural sunlight. It emits 10,000 lux of bright white light and features a sleek and modern design that can be adjusted to multiple angles. The Lumine Light Therapy Lamp is also lightweight and portable, making it easy to use at home or on the go.

4. Day-Light Sky Bright Light Therapy Lamp: The Day-Light Sky Bright Light Therapy Lamp is a powerful light therapy device that emits 10,000 lux of bright white light. It features a large, adjustable screen that can be angled to provide optimal light exposure, and it also includes a programmable timer and adjustable light intensity.

5. Theralite Aura Daylight Therapy Lamp: The Theralite Aura Daylight Therapy Lamp is a compact and portable light therapy device that is designed to help improve mood and energy levels. It emits 10,000 lux of bright white light and features a sleek and modern design. The Aura Daylight Therapy Lamp is also easy to use, with a simple on/off switch and adjustable brightness settings.

6. Lightphoria 10,000LUX Energy Light Lamp: The Lightphoria 10,000LUX Energy Light Lamp is a budget-friendly light therapy device that emits 10,000 lux of bright white light. It features a compact and portable design, making it easy to use at home or in the office. The

Lightphoria also includes adjustable brightness settings and a timer function.

7. Miroco Light Therapy Lamp: The Miroco Light Therapy Lamp is a versatile light therapy device that emits 10,000 lux of bright white light. It features a sleek and modern design, adjustable brightness settings, and a timer function. The Miroco Light Therapy Lamp is also portable, making it easy to use at home, in the office, or on the go.

In summary, there are many different light therapy devices available on the market, each with their own unique features and benefits. Some devices, such as the Verilux HappyLight and Circadian Optics Lumine Light Therapy Lamp, are designed to mimic natural sunlight, while others, such as the Philips SmartSleep Wake-Up Light and Theralite Aura Daylight Therapy Lamp, are designed to help regulate the body's natural wake-up cycle. Whether you are looking for a powerful and versatile light therapy device or a more budget-friendly option, there are many great options to choose from.

Chapter 6: Smart Pillows
How They Work and What They Offer

Smart pillows are the latest innovation in sleep technology. These pillows are designed to provide a comfortable sleeping experience while also tracking and monitoring your sleep habits. They come equipped with sensors, microphones, and other electronic components to gather data about your sleep patterns and provide feedback that can help you improve your sleep quality.

The basic function of smart pillows is to monitor your sleep cycle and provide information about the duration and quality of your sleep. They use sensors to detect movements and sounds, such as snoring, that may disrupt your sleep. Some smart pillows also offer features such as temperature control and adjustable firmness to provide maximum comfort and help you fall asleep faster.

Smart pillows are usually connected to a smartphone app that collects data about your sleep patterns and provides you with personalized recommendations for improving your sleep. The app may also include features such as meditation or relaxation exercises to help you fall asleep faster and sleep more deeply.

One popular feature of smart pillows is their ability to play soothing sounds or white noise to help you fall asleep.

Some smart pillows also come equipped with built-in speakers, allowing you to listen to music or other audio content without disturbing your sleeping partner.

Another feature that some smart pillows offer is an alarm that wakes you up gradually by slowly increasing the brightness of the pillow's lights or playing gentle sounds, such as birds chirping. This can help you wake up feeling more refreshed and less groggy.

Smart pillows also offer the convenience of being easy to clean, as many models come with removable covers that can be washed in a washing machine.

Overall, smart pillows offer a combination of comfort and technology to provide a personalized sleep experience. By monitoring your sleep patterns and providing feedback, they can help you make adjustments to your sleep habits and improve your overall sleep quality.

Pros and Cons

Smart pillows are an innovative solution that is aimed at improving sleep quality. They offer several benefits, but they also have some limitations. In this section, we'll discuss the pros and cons of smart pillows.

Pros:

1. Sleep monitoring: Smart pillows can monitor your sleep patterns and provide data on how long you slept, how many times you woke up, and other important metrics. This data can help you identify areas where you need to improve your sleep habits.

2. Comfort: Smart pillows are designed to provide maximum comfort while you sleep. They are made with materials that contour to your head and neck, which helps to alleviate pressure points and reduce pain.

3. Personalization: Some smart pillows offer personalized features such as adjustable height and firmness. This allows you to customize the pillow to your specific sleep needs, which can lead to better sleep.

4. Connectivity: Smart pillows can be connected to your phone or other devices, allowing you to control the pillow's settings and view your sleep data.

Cons:

1. Cost: Smart pillows can be quite expensive compared to traditional pillows. The added technology and features make them a premium product.

2. Power source: Most smart pillows require a power source, which means you need to charge them regularly. This can be inconvenient, especially if you forget to charge the pillow before going to bed.

3. Maintenance: Smart pillows require more maintenance than traditional pillows. The electronics inside the pillow need to be protected from moisture, and the cover needs to be removed and washed frequently.

4. Limited effectiveness: While smart pillows can provide useful sleep data, they may not be effective in addressing more serious sleep problems such as sleep apnea or chronic insomnia.

Overall, smart pillows are a great option for people who want to improve their sleep quality and are willing to invest in a premium product. They offer personalized features, sleep monitoring, and connectivity, but they also have some drawbacks such as cost and maintenance requirements.

Popular Pillows

Smart pillows have become increasingly popular in recent years, with a wide range of options available to consumers. Here are some of the most popular smart pillows on the market:

1. Moona Pillow: The Moona Pillow is designed to help regulate your body temperature as you sleep. It uses a water-based system to cool or warm the pillow to your desired temperature. The pillow also includes a sleep tracking sensor and can be controlled through a mobile app.

2. ZEEQ Smart Pillow: The ZEEQ Smart Pillow is a multifunctional pillow that includes sleep tracking, snoring detection, and music playback capabilities. The pillow's snoring detection feature will vibrate to encourage the sleeper to change their position to reduce snoring. The ZEEQ pillow can also be controlled through a mobile app.

3. Dreampad Pillow: The Dreampad Pillow is a pillow that includes built-in speakers that play music or white noise through the pillow itself. The pillow's sound vibrations are designed to help the sleeper relax and fall asleep faster. The Dreampad Pillow also includes a sleep tracking feature.

4. Withings Sleep Tracking Pad: The Withings Sleep Tracking Pad is not a pillow itself, but rather a pad that can be placed under any pillow. The pad includes sleep tracking

capabilities, as well as snoring detection and environmental monitoring. The Withings pad connects to a mobile app to provide detailed sleep data and insights.

5. Nitetronic Goodnite Anti-Snore Pillow: The Nitetronic Goodnite Anti-Snore Pillow is designed to reduce snoring. The pillow's built-in sensors can detect when the sleeper begins to snore, and the pillow will then gently adjust its height to encourage the sleeper to change positions and stop snoring. The Goodnite pillow can also be controlled through a mobile app.

6. Smart Nora Pillow Insert: The Smart Nora Pillow Insert is a device that can be inserted into any pillow. The device includes a microphone that can detect when the sleeper begins to snore, and it will then gently adjust the pillow to encourage the sleeper to change positions and stop snoring. The Smart Nora device can be controlled through a mobile app and includes sleep tracking features.

7. Eight Sleep Pod Pro: The Eight Sleep Pod Pro is a high-tech smart mattress that includes a built-in pillow top. The mattress includes sleep tracking, temperature regulation, and smart alarm features, among others. The Eight Sleep Pod Pro can be controlled through a mobile app and also includes voice control capabilities.

These are just a few examples of the many smart pillows available on the market today. Each pillow offers unique features and capabilities, so it's important to research and compare different options to find the one that best meets your individual needs and preferences.

Chapter 7: Sleep Sound Machines
How They Work and What They Offer

Sleep sound machines, also known as white noise machines or sound therapy machines, are electronic devices that produce soothing sounds to help people sleep better. The sounds can include nature sounds, ambient noise, white noise, or pink noise. These devices can be used to mask external sounds, such as traffic noise or snoring, or to create a relaxing atmosphere that promotes sleep. In this section, we will discuss how sleep sound machines work, the different types of sounds they offer, and how they can benefit your sleep.

How They Work

Sleep sound machines work by creating a background noise that masks other sounds, making it easier to fall asleep and stay asleep. They do this by producing a constant, low-level sound that is less distracting than sudden or irregular noises. The sound can be adjusted to your preferences, allowing you to choose the volume and type of sound that works best for you.

Most sleep sound machines use digital technology to produce the sounds, although some models use real sound recordings or analog technology. The sound can be played through built-in speakers or through headphones, depending on the model.

What They Offer

Sleep sound machines offer a variety of sounds to help you relax and sleep better. Here are some of the most common sounds offered by sleep sound machines:

1. Nature sounds: These can include the sound of rain, thunder, waves, birds, or a forest.

2. Ambient noise: This can include the sound of a fan, a humming air conditioner, or other subtle background noises.

3. White noise: This is a type of noise that contains all frequencies at equal intensity. It is often compared to the sound of static on a TV or radio.

4. Pink noise: This is a type of noise that is similar to white noise but has more power in the lower frequencies. It is often described as a "deep rumble" or "dull roar."

Sleep sound machines may also offer additional features, such as timers, alarms, or the ability to play music or other audio files.

Benefits of Sleep Sound Machines

Sleep sound machines have several benefits that can help improve the quality of your sleep. Here are some of the ways that sleep sound machines can benefit you:

1. Masking external sounds: Sleep sound machines can mask external sounds that may disrupt your sleep, such as traffic noise, snoring, or barking dogs.

2. Creating a relaxing atmosphere: The soothing sounds produced by sleep sound machines can create a relaxing atmosphere that promotes sleep and relaxation.

3. Reducing stress: The sounds produced by sleep sound machines can help reduce stress and promote relaxation.

4. Improving focus: Sleep sound machines can also be used to help improve focus and concentration, by creating a quiet and distraction-free environment.

5. Providing a consistent sleep environment: Sleep sound machines can help provide a consistent sleep environment, which is important for people who are sensitive to changes in their surroundings.

Conclusion

Sleep sound machines are a popular and effective way to improve the quality of your sleep. They work by creating a relaxing atmosphere that masks external sounds and promotes relaxation. With a variety of sounds to choose from, sleep sound machines can be customized to your preferences and needs. By using a sleep sound machine, you can enjoy the benefits of better sleep and wake up feeling refreshed and energized.

Pros and Cons

Sleep sound machines, also known as white noise machines or sound conditioners, have both advantages and disadvantages when it comes to improving sleep quality.

Pros:

1. Masking of Noise: Sleep sound machines can help to mask noise that might otherwise disturb sleep, such as traffic or loud neighbors. The steady, gentle sound of white noise or natural sounds like rain, waves or birds can create a soothing atmosphere and provide a sense of privacy.

2. Reduction of Stress: Sleep sound machines have been shown to reduce stress levels and promote relaxation, which can improve overall sleep quality. The calming sounds of nature or white noise can reduce cortisol levels, which is the hormone associated with stress.

3. Improving Focus: Sleep sound machines can also be used to help improve focus and concentration during the day. The sounds help to drown out distracting background noise and create a peaceful environment for work or studying.

4. Portable and Convenient: Sleep sound machines are portable and easy to use, which makes them a convenient tool for improving sleep quality both at home and while

travelling. They can be used in hotels, on airplanes, or anywhere else where noise might be a problem.

Cons:

1. Limited Effectiveness: While sleep sound machines can be effective in masking noise and creating a relaxing environment, they may not be sufficient for those with more severe sleep problems. The sounds may only be helpful to those who have minor disruptions to their sleep, such as occasional snoring or outside noise.

2. Habituation: Over time, some people may become habituated to the sound of the machine, making it less effective in helping them fall asleep. This means that they may need to increase the volume or change the type of sound to continue getting the benefits.

3. Sleep Disruptions: Sleep sound machines can also be a source of sleep disruptions, especially if they are too loud or if they produce sounds that are too high-pitched or too distracting. Some people may find the sound to be annoying, which can make it harder for them to fall asleep.

4. May Depend on Personal Preferences: The type of sound produced by sleep sound machines may depend on personal preferences. Some people may find certain types of sounds, such as white noise or nature sounds, to be more

relaxing than others. This means that finding the right sound for an individual may take some trial and error.

Overall, sleep sound machines can be a useful tool for improving sleep quality, particularly for those with mild sleep disruptions. However, they may not be effective for everyone, and personal preferences and individual needs should be taken into consideration when using these devices.

Popular Machines

In this section, we will explore sleep sound machines, a popular device used to promote relaxation and a peaceful sleep environment. We will discuss how they work, what they offer, and their pros and cons. We will also provide a list of popular machines on the market.

How They Work and What They Offer:

Sleep sound machines are designed to produce soothing sounds that help people relax and fall asleep. They work by producing different types of sound, including white noise, nature sounds, and ambient sounds.

White noise is a consistent and steady sound that helps mask other background noises, making it easier to fall asleep and stay asleep. It is often compared to the sound of a fan or an air conditioner. Nature sounds, on the other hand, are recorded sounds of the natural environment, such as rainfall, ocean waves, and birds singing. These sounds can be very calming and relaxing, helping people drift off to sleep.

Ambient sounds are a combination of different types of sounds, including white noise and nature sounds. Some sleep sound machines allow users to customize the sounds by adjusting the volume and the type of sound. Some even have a feature that simulates a heartbeat to help people feel more relaxed.

Sleep sound machines offer several benefits to users. They can create a peaceful sleep environment, reduce distractions, and improve sleep quality. They can also be helpful for people who have trouble falling asleep due to anxiety, stress, or other factors.

Pros and Cons:

There are several benefits to using sleep sound machines, but there are also some drawbacks to consider.

Pros:

1. Creates a peaceful sleep environment: Sleep sound machines produce calming sounds that help create a peaceful sleep environment. They can mask other background noises and make it easier to fall asleep.

2. Reduces distractions: Sleep sound machines can help reduce distractions that can interfere with sleep, such as traffic noise, noisy neighbors, or barking dogs.

3. Improves sleep quality: By promoting relaxation and reducing distractions, sleep sound machines can help improve sleep quality and help users wake up feeling more refreshed.

4. Helps manage anxiety and stress: Sleep sound machines can be helpful for people who have trouble falling asleep due to anxiety or stress.

Cons:

1. May not be effective for everyone: While sleep sound machines can be effective for many people, they may not work for everyone. Some people may find the sounds annoying or distracting.

2. May become a sleep association: Over time, some people may become dependent on sleep sound machines to fall asleep, making it difficult to sleep without one.

3. Requires electricity: Sleep sound machines require electricity, so they may not be suitable for camping or other situations where electricity is not available.

Popular Machines:

There are many sleep sound machines on the market, each with its unique features and benefits. Here are some of the most popular machines:

1. LectroFan: The LectroFan is a compact, portable sleep sound machine that offers ten different fan sounds and ten different white noise sounds. It is easy to use and has a timer feature that can be set for up to eight hours.

2. Marpac Dohm Classic: The Marpac Dohm Classic is a popular sleep sound machine that produces a consistent and soothing sound that mimics the sound of a fan. It is easy to use, durable, and produces a sound that is comfortable for most users.

3. Adaptive Sound Technologies LectroFan Evo: The Adaptive Sound Technologies LectroFan Evo is a versatile sleep sound machine that offers twenty different unique sounds, including white noise, nature sounds, and fan sounds. It has a compact design, making it easy to travel with, and offers a timer feature.

4. Yogasleep Dohm Uno: The Yogasleep Dohm Uno is a compact and affordable sleep sound machine that has gained a lot of popularity in recent years. It features a two-speed motor that produces the signature "white noise" sound that is known to promote relaxation and restful sleep. The Dohm Uno has a simple design with just an on/off switch and a volume control, making it easy to use and operate.

One of the standout features of the Dohm Uno is its compact size. It is small enough to fit in the palm of your hand, making it an ideal travel companion. Its small size also means it can fit easily on a nightstand or a desk, without taking up too much space. Despite its small size, the Dohm Uno still produces a powerful sound that can effectively mask unwanted noises and help you fall asleep faster.

Another advantage of the Dohm Uno is its affordability. It is one of the most budget-friendly sleep sound machines on the market, making it accessible to a wide range of people. Its low price point doesn't compromise on its quality or effectiveness, making it a great option for those who want to try out a sleep sound machine without investing a lot of money.

However, like any product, the Dohm Uno has some downsides. The lack of a timer feature can be inconvenient for some users who want to set it to turn off after a certain period of time. Additionally, the limited sound options might not appeal to those who prefer a variety of sounds to choose from.

Despite these drawbacks, the Yogasleep Dohm Uno has been well received by customers, and its popularity is a testament to its effectiveness and value for money.

Chapter 8: Comparing and Contrasting Methods
Summary of Pros and Cons

In this chapter, we will compare and contrast the different sleep technologies that we have discussed in the previous chapters. Each sleep technology has its unique features, advantages, and disadvantages that make it stand out from the others. In this section, we will provide a summary of the pros and cons of each sleep technology to help you choose the best sleep solution that meets your needs.

Sleep Trackers Pros:

- Provide comprehensive sleep data, including sleep stages, duration, and quality

- Allow for personalized sleep recommendations

- May motivate individuals to adopt healthier sleep habits

- Can detect sleep disorders

Cons:

- May cause anxiety and stress if users obsess over the data

- Data may not be 100% accurate

- Expensive models may not be affordable for some users

- Some users may find wearing a sleep tracker uncomfortable

Smart Mattresses Pros:

- Provide customized sleep experiences for couples with different sleep preferences
- Can adjust firmness, temperature, and elevation to promote better sleep
- May detect snoring and adjust to prevent it
- Can provide detailed sleep data through an app

Cons:

- Expensive compared to traditional mattresses
- Require a power source, which may be inconvenient
- Limited customization options for single sleepers
- Some users may find the technology intrusive

Sleep Apps Pros:

- Accessible and affordable
- Provide a wide range of sleep solutions, including guided meditations and relaxing music
- May provide sleep analysis and recommendations
- Can be used on a mobile device for on-the-go use

Cons:

- May not be as accurate as other sleep technologies
- Can drain the battery life of mobile devices

- Overuse of devices before bedtime may affect sleep quality

- Some apps may have hidden fees or require a subscription

White Noise Machines Pros:

- Can provide a calming and relaxing sleep environment

- May help reduce background noise that can disrupt sleep

- Can be customized to meet individual preferences

- Can be portable and affordable

Cons:

- May not work for everyone

- Can be distracting or irritating for some users

- Limited sound options may not appeal to all users

- May not address underlying sleep problems

Light Therapy Devices Pros:

- May help regulate circadian rhythms and improve sleep

- Can help alleviate symptoms of seasonal affective disorder (SAD)

- May improve mood and energy levels

- Some devices can also function as alarm clocks

Cons:

- Expensive compared to other sleep technologies

- May require significant time commitment and adherence to a schedule

- Some devices may cause eye strain or other side effects

- May not work for all individuals

Smart Pillows Pros:

- Can adjust to individual preferences for firmness and support

- May help prevent snoring and other sleep disruptions

- Can provide detailed sleep data through an app

- Can be portable and easy to use

Cons:

- Expensive compared to traditional pillows

- May not be comfortable for all users

- May require power, which may be inconvenient

- May not address underlying sleep problems

Sleep Sound Machines Pros:

- Can create a calming sleep environment

- May help reduce stress and anxiety

- Can be customized to meet individual preferences

- Can be portable and affordable

Cons:

- May not work for everyone
- Limited sound options may not appeal to all users
- May not address underlying sleep problems
- Some users may find the technology intrusive

In conclusion, each sleep technology has its unique strengths and weaknesses. The best sleep solution for you will depend on your personal preferences, needs, and budget. It's important to consider the pros and cons of each technology and to choose the one that fits your lifestyle and promotes healthy sleep habits. With the wide range of sleep technologies available today, it's easier than ever to find a sleep solution that works for you.

Ultimately, the decision on which sleep technology to use will depend on your specific needs and circumstances. For those who struggle with falling asleep or staying asleep due to noise or environmental factors, a white noise machine or a sleep sound machine may be the best option. Those who struggle with regulating their sleep schedule may find light therapy devices to be helpful, while others who experience discomfort during sleep may benefit from a smart mattress. Sleep apps and smart pillows can be useful for those who prefer a more technological approach to improving their sleep.

It's important to keep in mind that while technology can be helpful in promoting healthy sleep, it's not a substitute for healthy sleep habits. This includes maintaining a regular sleep schedule, avoiding stimulants before bedtime, creating a comfortable sleep environment, and engaging in relaxation techniques before bed. Additionally, it's important to consult with a healthcare provider if you have ongoing sleep issues or underlying medical conditions that may be affecting your sleep.

In the end, the key to finding the right sleep technology is to do your research, consider your personal preferences and needs, and be willing to try different options until you find what works best for you. With the wide range of sleep technologies available today, it's easier than ever to improve your sleep quality and overall health.

Criteria for Comparison

When it comes to comparing and contrasting different sleep technologies, it is important to consider various criteria to determine which one might be the best fit for you. The following are some of the key factors that you may want to keep in mind when evaluating different sleep technologies.

1. Effectiveness: One of the primary considerations for any sleep technology is whether it actually works. Does it help you fall asleep more easily, stay asleep longer, and wake up feeling more refreshed? You'll want to look at factors such as the type of technology, the specific features that it offers, and any research or studies that have been conducted on its effectiveness.

2. Comfort: Another important factor to consider is how comfortable a sleep technology is to use. For example, a mattress or pillow that is too hard or too soft might not be supportive enough for your body, leading to discomfort and disrupted sleep. Similarly, a light therapy device that is too bright or too harsh could be unpleasant to use, making it less likely that you will stick with it over time.

3. Customization: Many sleep technologies offer a range of features and settings that can be customized to your individual needs. For example, a white noise machine might offer different types of sounds or adjustable volume levels. A

sleep app might allow you to set a personalized sleep schedule or track your sleep data. The more customizable a technology is, the more likely it is to meet your specific needs and preferences.

4. Ease of Use: Some sleep technologies are easier to use than others. A mattress or pillow, for example, is relatively straightforward to set up and use. A sleep app might require more initial setup and customization, but can be easier to use over time. A complex sleep sound machine or light therapy device might take more time to figure out, but can be worth it if the benefits are significant.

5. Price: Sleep technologies can range from very affordable to quite expensive. For many people, price is an important consideration when choosing a sleep solution. You'll want to balance the benefits of a given technology against its cost, as well as consider how long it is likely to last and whether it is worth the investment.

6. Safety: Safety is also an important consideration when choosing a sleep technology. You'll want to look for products that are certified by recognized organizations and that have been tested for safety. Additionally, you should be aware of any potential risks associated with a given technology, such as possible side effects or interactions with medications.

7. Durability: Finally, it's important to consider the durability of a sleep technology. Some products, such as mattresses or pillows, may need to be replaced every few years to maintain their effectiveness. Other technologies, such as sleep apps, can be updated with new features over time. When evaluating a sleep technology, consider how long it is likely to last and whether it is worth the investment.

Overall, there are many different factors to consider when comparing and contrasting sleep technologies. By keeping these criteria in mind, you can better evaluate which sleep solution might be the best fit for your individual needs and preferences.

Recommendations for Different Needs

Choosing the right sleep technology can be a daunting task, especially with the wide range of options available. Here are some recommendations for different needs to help you make an informed decision:

1. For those who have trouble falling asleep:

- Sleep apps can be a great tool for those who have trouble falling asleep. They often offer guided meditations, relaxing sounds, and other features that can help you relax and unwind before bed.

- A white noise machine or sleep sound machine can also be effective in blocking out distractions and creating a soothing environment for sleep.

2. For those who have trouble staying asleep:

- A smart mattress can monitor your sleep and adjust the firmness and position to keep you comfortable and asleep throughout the night.

- A smart pillow can detect snoring and adjust its position to prevent it, helping you stay asleep.

3. For those who have trouble waking up:

- A light therapy device can simulate a sunrise and help regulate your circadian rhythm, making it easier to wake up naturally and feeling more refreshed.

- A smart alarm clock can wake you up with gentle vibrations, rather than a jarring noise, which can be less disruptive and more pleasant.

4. For those who travel frequently:

- A portable white noise machine or sleep sound machine can be a great tool for creating a familiar sleep environment, no matter where you are.

- Sleep apps are also a great option, as they can be used on your phone or tablet, making it easy to use them on the go.

5. For those on a budget:

- A simple white noise machine or sleep sound machine can be an affordable option for creating a soothing sleep environment.

- Sleep apps are often free or have low subscription fees, making them a budget-friendly option.

6. For those with a partner who has different sleep preferences:

- A smart mattress with dual firmness settings can accommodate different sleep preferences for each partner.

- A white noise machine or sleep sound machine can mask noise and create a peaceful sleep environment for both partners.

It's important to remember that the best sleep solution for you will depend on your personal preferences, needs, and budget. These recommendations can serve as a starting point for finding the right sleep technology to help you get the best quality sleep possible.

Conclusion

Recap of Importance of Good Sleep

Sleep is an essential part of our lives, and getting a good night's sleep is crucial for our physical and mental well-being. However, with the stresses of modern life and the prevalence of technology, many people struggle to get the quality and quantity of sleep they need. In this book, we have explored various sleep technologies and methods to help improve the quality of our sleep. But before we conclude, let's recap why getting good sleep is so important.

Sleep is critical for our physical health. During sleep, the body carries out vital processes that help to repair and rejuvenate the body. For example, sleep is essential for the immune system to fight off infections and inflammation. Chronic sleep deprivation can lead to a weakened immune system, making us more susceptible to illness.

Sleep is also crucial for our mental health. It plays a crucial role in cognitive processes, such as attention, memory, and learning. Lack of sleep can lead to a decline in cognitive function and can make it difficult to concentrate, make decisions, and even affect our mood. Chronic sleep deprivation can also contribute to the development of mental health disorders, such as anxiety and depression.

Additionally, good sleep is essential for maintaining a healthy weight. Sleep plays a role in regulating hormones that control appetite and metabolism. Lack of sleep can disrupt these hormones, leading to an increased risk of obesity and related health problems.

It's clear that good sleep is essential for our overall health and well-being. Therefore, it's crucial to prioritize healthy sleep habits, such as maintaining a consistent sleep schedule, creating a sleep-conducive environment, and avoiding technology before bed. In addition, incorporating sleep technologies, such as sleep apps, white noise machines, light therapy devices, smart pillows, and sleep sound machines, can also be beneficial in promoting better sleep.

Overall, the importance of good sleep cannot be overstated. It's a fundamental aspect of our lives that impacts our physical, mental, and emotional health. By prioritizing healthy sleep habits and incorporating sleep technologies, we can all work towards achieving better quality sleep and improving our overall well-being.

Final Thoughts and Recommendations

As we've seen, there are many different sleep technologies available to help us get a good night's sleep. Each technology has its unique strengths and weaknesses, and the best solution for you will depend on your individual needs, preferences, and budget. However, there are some general recommendations that can help guide you in choosing the right sleep technology for you.

First, it's important to prioritize sleep and make it a part of your daily routine. This means going to bed and waking up at the same time every day, even on weekends. It also means creating a relaxing sleep environment, which can be aided by sleep technologies such as white noise machines, light therapy devices, and smart pillows.

Second, it's important to address any underlying health issues that may be interfering with your sleep. If you suspect that you have a sleep disorder such as sleep apnea, it's important to see a healthcare professional for diagnosis and treatment. Sleep technologies can be helpful in managing some sleep disorders, but they are not a substitute for professional medical care.

Third, it's important to choose sleep technologies that are safe and effective. Look for technologies that have been scientifically validated and are backed by research. Consider the reputation of the manufacturer and read reviews from other users to get a sense of their experience with the technology.

Fourth, consider the cost of the technology and whether it fits within your budget. While some technologies can be expensive, others are relatively affordable. Don't assume that the most expensive technology is necessarily the best. Consider what you can realistically afford and what will provide the most benefit for your needs.

Finally, keep in mind that sleep technologies are not a magic solution for poor sleep. They can be a helpful tool in promoting healthy sleep habits, but they should be used in combination with other strategies such as exercise, healthy eating, and stress reduction techniques.

In conclusion, the importance of good sleep cannot be overstated. It's essential for physical health, mental well-being, and overall quality of life. Sleep technologies can be a helpful tool in promoting healthy sleep habits, but they should be chosen and used wisely. By prioritizing sleep, addressing any underlying health issues, choosing safe and effective sleep technologies, and combining them with other healthy habits, we can all get the restful, restorative sleep that we need to thrive.

THE END

Potential References

Introduction:

National Sleep Foundation. (n.d.). Why is sleep important? https://www.sleepfoundation.org/articles/why-sleep-important

American Sleep Association. (n.d.). Sleep statistics. https://www.sleepassociation.org/sleep/sleep-statistics/

Sleep Cycle. (n.d.). About Sleep Cycle. https://www.sleepcycle.com/about/

Chapter 1: Sleep Trackers

Sleep Foundation. (2021). Sleep tracking. https://www.sleepfoundation.org/sleep-tracking

SleepScore Labs. (n.d.). How it works. https://www.sleepscore.com/how-it-works/

PLOS One. (2018). Validity of sleep trackers for estimating sleep: A systematic review and meta-analysis. https://journals.plos.org/plosone/article?id=10.1371/journal.pone.0209485

Chapter 2: Smart Mattresses

The Sleep Judge. (n.d.). What is a smart mattress? https://www.thesleepjudge.com/what-is-a-smart-mattress/

Sleep Number. (n.d.). How it works. https://www.sleepnumber.com/how-it-works

Consumer Reports. (2021). Best mattresses of 2021. https://www.consumerreports.org/mattresses/best-mattresses-of-the-year/

Chapter 3: Sleep Apps

Sleep Foundation. (2021). Sleep apps. https://www.sleepfoundation.org/sleep-tools-tips/sleep-apps

Healthline. (2019). 10 of the best sleep apps for tracking and improving your sleep. https://www.healthline.com/health/best-sleep-tracking-apps

National Sleep Foundation. (n.d.). The science of sleep. https://www.sleepfoundation.org/sleep-science

Chapter 4: White Noise Machines

Sound Oasis. (n.d.). About white noise. https://www.soundoasis.com/pages/about-white-noise

American Tinnitus Association. (n.d.). Sound therapy. https://www.ata.org/managing-tinnitus/treatment-options/sound-therapy

Healthline. (2021). The 8 best sound machines of 2021. https://www.healthline.com/health/best-sound-machines

Chapter 5: Light Therapy Devices

Mayo Clinic. (2019). Light therapy. https://www.mayoclinic.org/tests-procedures/light-therapy/about/pac-20384604

National Institute of Mental Health. (2019). Seasonal Affective Disorder. https://www.nimh.nih.gov/health/topics/seasonal-affective-disorder/index.shtml

Philips. (n.d.). How light therapy works. https://www.usa.philips.com/c-m-pe/light-therapy/how-light-therapy-works

Chapter 6: Smart Pillows

Sleep Number. (n.d.). What is a smart pillow? https://www.sleepnumber.com/smart-pillow

CNET. (2021). Best smart pillows for 2021. https://www.cnet.com/home/smart-home/best-smart-pillows/

Sleep.org. (n.d.). The science of sleep. https://www.sleep.org/the-science-of-sleep/

Chapter 7: Sleep Sound Machines

"The Science of Sleep: Understanding What Happens When You Sleep" by Wallace B. Mendelson, M.D., published by A Johns Hopkins Press Health Book

"The Best Sound Machines for a Better Night's Sleep" by Emily Shiffer, published by Men's Health

"How White Noise Machines Can Help You Sleep Better and Live Healthier" by Paige Smith, published by Prevention

Chapter 8: Comparing and Contrasting Methods

"Comparing Sleep Tracking Methods" by Sarah Tew, published by CNET

"The Best Sleep Technology for a Good Night's Sleep" by Meghan Rabbitt, published by Consumer Reports

"A Sleep Expert Reviews Popular Devices That Claim to Improve Sleep" by Dr. Rajkumar Dasgupta, published by Sleep Foundation

Conclusion

"Sleep Smarter: 21 Essential Strategies to Sleep Your Way to a Better Body, Better Health, and Bigger Success" by Shawn Stevenson, published by Rodale Books

"Why We Sleep: Unlocking the Power of Sleep and Dreams" by Matthew Walker, published by Scribner

"Sleep Revolution: Transforming Your Life, One Night at a Time" by Arianna Huffington, published by Harmony Books

www.ingramcontent.com/pod-product-compliance
Lightning Source LLC
LaVergne TN
LVHW012126070526
838202LV00056B/5868